MEDITERRANEAN

DIET

✳✳✳

A Practical Guide to the Food
Wisdom of the Mediterranean

JUDITH ELLEN PERRY

This book is solely for educational and informational purposes and should not be regarded as a substitute for the medical advice or care of physicians or medical professionals. Since each person is unique, the services of an appropriate medical professional should be sought for any health situation or question. The author and the publisher specifically disclaim responsibility for any adverse effects allegedly arising from the application or use of the information and advice in this book.

Contents

Chapter 1. How I Became Interested in Mediterranean Diet

I had the gratifying experience of finding my own special Greek island. For twenty years I had been living and teaching in Athens, the capital, deeply entering a Mediterranean lifestyle, but without thinking about it consciously. Then I discovered Skyros, an island in the Aegean. Some friends of mine frequented the island to collect folk woodcarvings and often invited me along.

I fell in love with Skyros and the poetry of its landscape: the pure and clear outline of the rocky offshore islets against the turquoise sea, the dolphins making their way to the sheltered bays at sunset, the Milky Way, bright enough at night to read by. The colors were extraordinary: the silvery green of olive groves set against the deep blue sky, the white of the limed villages clustered on the hillside, the lichen-flecked gray of ancient fortress walls. Each time of day had its own activity: the fishing boats returning at dawn to unload their catch and mend their nets, the wild goats congregating in the shade of plane trees in the heat of the day, the gathering of friends on a grapevine-covered terrace overlooking the sea at dusk to exchange the news of the day, and the cuckoos and owls emerging at night in the pine forest to begin their calls.

Each season also had its own joy—spring brought fields of red poppies, newborn lambs, and the full week of Easter preparations and rituals. Summer was fishing for octopus, the fragrance of night blooming flowers, and the purple-stained hands and clothes sported at mulberry-gathering time. Fall was the time for gathering wild thyme and oregano, being dressed in the traditional costume by the women of Skyros, and dancing local circle dances in the main square. Winter was the wooden boats hugging the shore very close as they made their way in stormy weather, the pomegranate bushes full of big Christmas ornament-sized pomegranates that turned red just at Christmas time, and learning to weave while sitting near the fire. But above all there were the people of the island, with their warmth and hospitality and their humane spirit.

I had arrived on Skyros at a crucial time. It had been one of the most isolated of islands, accessible only by the small open boats called caiques that sailed without scheduled service—only when hired and only in good weather. When I first arrived the food system on Skyros still retained many traditional ways, even as other islands with better transportation links had started to change dietary habits decades earlier. Then, after much discussion, the inhabitants of Skyros purchased their own communal ferryboat, and suddenly there was a daily all-weather connection with the mainland. With the ferry connection, the traditional food ways on Skyros Island would likely come under considerable pressure, as had been the pattern on other islands. It was possible the ancient system would vanish.

I realized a valuable tradition was slated for change, but much still remained. I wanted to learn as much about it as possible while I still could. I visited a local family I had met through my friends. I was able to visit for several weeks at a time at different seasons over a period of several years. My Greek was just serviceable enough to give me the privilege of observing and understanding time-hallowed patterns of food preparation and eating. I contemplated how to make the traditional foodways more known, how to communicate the spirit and attitudes that underlie them, the way the diet is actually lived by the Mediterraneans themselves, and the joy and satisfaction of it.

I began offering seminars at my home in Athens, attended mostly by northern European tourists who found the Mediterranean way of life attractive and wanted to learn more about it. The Mediterranean combines many enticing features. It remains a natural civilization, retaining its closeness to nature, something that is fast receding in many other places. It is a civilization of the sun, with the climatic and scenic beauty that implies. It also has among the deepest historical roots, and is thus informed by ancient, rich traditions and cultures. There is nothing quite like this combination.

The result is not only a diet but also a lifestyle that has been fine-tuned over the centuries by and for many people. It relies on the time-tested health, taste, and food preparation experience of millions of people.

I took notice when research began showing just how comprehensive the health benefits of the Mediterranean diet are. Through epidemiological studies and randomized trials, the evidence of benefits is growing. The good news about the positive health outcomes of the Mediterranean diet has, for me, an incredible implication. One of the most desirable, delicious, and enjoyable ways of eating ever conceived, is a path of health and wellness. That is something to really sit up and take notice of.

This lifestyle and diet have endured because they have generated wellbeing and have been fine tuned over many generations. This gives us confidence in the safety and practicality of the diet. Contrast this situation with the almost spectacular misinformation and conflicting information on the subject of nutrition often seen nowadays. This misinformation not only emanates from those with economic interests, but also from experts and government agencies. It is so pervasive that it has become necessary to clear our minds of preconceived attitudes and lift ourselves above the morass. The two thousand year track record of the Mediterranean diet gives us some confidence as we seek guidance.

Greece could be considered a prime area for studying the Mediterranean diet. Historically, it is one of the diet's points of origin, and as the Greeks colonized the Mediterranean in ancient times their way of eating was spread. Some of the original modern work on the health effects of the diet was done in Greece. In addition, Greece, especially the Aegean islands, has retained the traditional diet more than many other countries of the region.

During the time I lived in Greece, I also traveled throughout the Mediterranean. I was able to observe much variation in the cuisine. For example, some countries cook with olives, while in others olives are a separate side dish and never a part of a cooked dish. Some countries use more oil in their cooking than others. (I have eaten fried eggs in Sicily where the olive oil came up over the eggs!)

In spite of its culinary diversity, the Mediterranean has shared climate and agricultural conditions. These relatively dry conditions foster deep-rooted plants such as olive trees and grapevines and discourage large animal grazing. Because of this, the basic ingredients have traditionally been the same throughout the region, as are the basic dietary principles.

What is the Mediterranean Diet?

The Greek diet of the 1950s was originally considered the quintessential Mediterranean diet. The meaning of the term has now evolved so that it is a construct, a construct of proven healthy eating that doesn't necessarily exist in any one country. It mirrors a traditional pattern of eating that people around the Mediterranean Sea have followed for thousands of years. It emphasizes unprocessed foods, especially vegetables, fruits, fish, beans, whole grains, nuts, and olive oil. It minimizes red meat (that is, beef, pork, and lamb), dairy products, and sweets. Low to moderate wine consumption is encompassed.

The Mediterranean diet is low in saturated fat from animal products, but it is not overall a low fat diet. Mostly due to its inclusion of nuts and olive oil, it is a medium fat diet. However, notice that these are relatively unrefined fats. One ground rule to always keep in mind is that the quality and source of fats is of prime importance. Refined fats, trans fats, and animal fats are minimized. The preponderance of fat in the diet comes from olive oil, fatty fish, and nuts.

In defining a Mediterranean diet, several recent studies have quantified the specific amounts of key ingredients:

3 to 4 Tablespoons a day olive oil

3 servings a week fish and seafood, with an emphasis on fatty fish

3 servings a week beans

2 servings a day vegetables, about 1 cup each, often one with lunch and one with dinner

3 servings a day fresh, whole fruit, one with breakfast, then as either a snack or as dessert with meals

3 servings a week nuts

1 glass of wine a day is optional

For those who have eaten out in Italian restaurants, a popular misconception is that it is a cheese and tomato or a pasta diet. Actually, the cuisine of current U.S. Italian, Spanish, or Greek restaurants does not match an authentic Mediterranean diet.

Advantages of the Mediterranean Diet

The health benefits are most impressive, and the evidence for them is increasingly compelling. The health secret of the Mediterranean diet is above all balance. The number one factor for health is that it has fewer foods that cause inflammation and more antioxidants and omega 3s that fight it. For detailed information on the health effects of the diet see the comprehensive review of medical literature in the bibliography and medical appendix of *The New Mediterranean Diet Cookbook* by Nancy Harmon Jenkins. In addition, the Health Letters of Tufts University, Harvard University, and the University of California, Berkeley, provide ongoing coverage of the most recent research. (See Further Reading at the end of the book for these.) However, I would like to present a few salient, general points.

The diet is associated with increased longevity, lower death rates from all causes, and lower rates of chronic disease. Earlier studies had reported findings that "meta-analysis of studies encompassing a total of nearly 1.6 million individuals shows that adherence to the eating pattern known as the Mediterranean diet significantly reduces mortality as well as the rates of various illnesses. These results seem to be clinically relevant for public health, in particular for encouraging a Mediterranean-like dietary pattern for primary prevention of major chronic diseases." (*Clinical Advisor*, November 2008 p. 19).

A study published in February 2013 in the *New England Journal of Medicine* extended these findings, reporting on a large study in Spain that linked Mediterranean diet to a significantly reduced risk of heart and circulatory disorders.

New knowledge of the health effects is coming in at an increasing pace. One impressive finding is that switching to a Mediterranean-style diet improves blood lipids quite rapidly, within a matter of weeks.

An important point about this way of eating, as a preventative, is that it is comprehensive and covers the whole body, not just targeting one or two body systems. Other, more specialized diets and regimens do accomplish certain specific nutritional and health goals, but at the cost of harm to health in other ways. As an example, certain extremely low fat diets may help the circulatory system but have been shown to add new risks, such as depression or early brain aging if followed for many years. The Mediterranean diet is a more comprehensive, holistic approach that does not benefit some systems of the body at the expense of others. This whole body aspect of the diet is also reflected by its association with such varied factors as bone health, lowered risk of depression, and stable blood sugar levels.

Those who begin to eat this way notice increases in day-to-day wellbeing. The healthy fats, sufficient protein, and whole grains encourage a dependable, steady flow of physical and mental energy through the day.

Holistic, positive effects on health are not the only story. Mediterranean diet also scores relatively well on ecological sustainability. A graph of the effect on the environment of various dietary constituents from the journal *Environmental Science and Technology* shows that oils, fruit, vegetables, cereals, chicken, and eggs rate relatively high in terms of environmental sustainability. Red meat and dairy products rate significantly lower. Olive oil rates much higher than seed oils.

In the Mediterranean diet, the foods with the most negative impact on the environment tend to be the ones least eaten, and the foods with minimum impact are the ones commonly eaten. This is in part because, as will be discussed shortly, the Mediterraneans eat meat relatively sparingly; in other words, the bulk of their food consumption comes from lower on the food chain. The fish commonly consumed also tend to be the smaller fish that are lower on oceanic food chains, and are thus, compared to species higher up the chain, lower in mercury and more sustainable. They are also caught closer to shore, using less invasive methods and expending less fuel.

As it is a general pattern of eating, the Mediterranean diet is flexible. It is a traditional pattern rather than meal plans, grams, and calorie counts. Most diets are regimented, interventionist diets. On a regimen, you need to become a true believer who thinks this diet will solve all your problems. The Mediterranean diet is more relaxed. You don't rely on the emotional high of committing to a new regimen, only to be unable to sustain the excitement and commitment after the initial emotional energy falters. The guidelines recognize that dietary needs vary by individual, and that individual needs can vary over time.

Biological individuality is crucial when it comes to diet. For example, individuals differ with respect to the optimum amount of oil in their diet, even if it is olive oil. (Perhaps we can look forward to a day when metabolic or genetic testing will become available to help us more effectively tailor our diets.) The Mediterranean diet can accommodate vegetarians or non-vegetarians. Protein is highly valued, but there are plenty of non-meat ways to get it. There are many vegetarian main dishes that are a part of daily eating.

Interestingly, the Mediterranean diet can accommodate those who enjoy cooking complex dishes, simple dishes, or even those who do very little cooking. It is more about food choices and attitudes than it is about cooking.

In its relaxed attitude, the diet asserts that there is no one ideal food or way of eating. Food is a profound subject that reaches into every part of life. This means that perfection cannot be found. We can only resolve to learn and experience more, start with a few small changes, and persevere.

Finally, the Mediterranean diet is a pleasure. The joy of food is the system's most basic underlying principle. It is a return to the most basic satisfactions: the joy of the first bite, the idea that food is precious, the notion that food can work its magic on us and our mood, or bind closer a group that eats together. The Mediterranean diet is the improver of health that adds pleasure to life. It is the healthy diet that seems more of a pleasure regimen than a health regimen.

Chapter 2. Food Choices: Meat and Meat Alternatives

As early as the ancient period, Mediterraneans had a distinctive point of view about meat products. Red meat was considered to have a dual nature. On the one hand, when taken in small amounts, it is considered a tonic and valuable for both immune strength and robust metabolism. It was especially important for children, and in older people it was felt to reduce bone fractures. On the other hand, it has been long believed that red meat leaves more waste material in the body than other foods, and this is true of even naturally raised meat. Modern science might offer the explanation that meat contains fatty acids that promote inflammation.

In spite of this, there is no feeling that red meat should be excluded completely from the diet. Protein is extremely highly valued—the word "protein" itself comes from a Greek word denoting "first in importance." As happens in every country with rising living standards, meat consumption has been increasing in the Mediterranean. In the Greek islands I saw that the only change wanted in the diet was a bit more meat on the table. The traditional way of eating was beloved, and fast food, packaged food, or new kinds of foods were not wanted. But meat a little more often was important, and that one change did happen.

Nevertheless, it is commonly believed that meat must be limited even when it can be afforded. The basic principle is that some valuable foods are only needed in small amounts—and more is not necessarily better.

Three main guidelines help with this:

(i) The most important thing is to limit portions to 2 to 4 ounces at a time, 10 to 12 ounces a week. A 16 ounce steakhouse portion is too much. Recipes that stretch meat, such as vegetables stuffed with a small amount of spiced meat, have been a part of Mediterranean cuisine for thousands of years.

For one used to eating larger amounts, a crucial point is to fill in the gap by eating something besides more salads and grains. The body is hard to fool and senses that protein and fat are missing. The gap should be filled by other rich foods, like eggs, nuts, beans, and olive oil.

(ii) Use certain strategies to garner the advantages of red meat while reducing its harmful effects.

a. Marinate the meat before cooking.

b. Use long, moist cooking at low temperatures, such as braised dishes. This is thought to make the meat more digestible and the protein more easily assimilated so one can get the benefits of meat while eating less of it.

c. Cook the meat with herbs and spices. Research has shown that seasonings such as oregano, rosemary, garlic, and cumin substantially reduce lipid oxidation when eaten with meat.

Scattering a teaspoon of capers over cooked meat has a similar effect. Capers are the antioxidant-filled bud of a Mediterranean plant; they are often used as a garnish. They are available brined in jars and are rinsed and patted dry before serving to reduce the salt.

d. Eat meat with a lot of vegetables and fiber. It is a matter of proportion. The Mediterraneans do not banish meat from the table; they only counsel that an equal or larger amount of vegetables should be eaten in the same meal. This strikes the right balance between drivers of inflammation, like saturated fat in red meat, and anti-inflammatory components of the meal, while at the same time providing enough protein.

e. Accompany the meal with beverages or garnishes that provide anti-oxidants. One way is to drink a moderate amount of red wine along with the meat—

not before or after. The simultaneous pairing of meat and wine is considered important—both should reside in the stomach at the same time. The point seems to be to make antioxidants available in the stomach at just the right time. (This is in line with studies showing that timing is a key issue with dietary antioxidants.) Also, since antioxidants are not stored in the body, frequent replenishment is required, preferably at each meal.

For those who do not take alcohol, there are many effective alternatives often used as a garnish. Lemon juice is often squeezed over the meat. Small slices of lemon only give a drop or two, not enough, so lemon halves are generally on the table at any Mediterranean meal. Pushing the tines of a fork into a lemon half and then squeezing the half around the fork will produce more juice without getting it on the fingers.

In addition to the dried herbs mentioned above that are used in cooking, fresh herbs are also used as a garnish, added after cooking is complete. The most important is flat-leaf parsley, which is cut with a kitchen shears and scattered over food. Fresh anise is also widely used.

(iii) Don't eat meat every day. The meatless Monday trend goes in the right direction. Similarly, it is well known that a Lenten type fast from meat in the early spring was traditional, although this is often abbreviated now to a few days.

By "red meat" the Mediterraneans usually mean beef, veal, pork, lamb, goat, and four-footed game such as venison. So, pork, ham, and bacon, sometimes advertised as "the other white meat," are considered red meat.

Eating Less Meat

If meat is reduced, a crucial question is what will replace it. In the Mediterranean diet, it is compensated for partially by increased con-sumption of vegetables and fruits, but this is by no means all. An important principle is the broad array of foods—eggs, fish, shellfish, organ meats, beans, nuts, and olive oil-rich dishes—that are used as alternatives to red meat. There has been a tendency to substitute mainly chicken for red meat in contemporary diets, and of course chicken can be a valid option, but in the Mediterranean it is considered just one of many.

This variety of alternatives to red meat is a crucial feature of the Mediterranean diet. The alternatives come close to red meat in calorie count and appetite satisfaction qualities, due to their oil and protein content.

Compare this situation to the well-known problem with many low fat diets—that in order to maintain the food's palatability and satisfaction qualities, the dropped fat calories are replaced by large amounts of carbohydrates. This throws off the body's metabolism, leading to new problems.

Let us now discuss individually some of the popular alternatives to red meat in the Mediterranean diet.

Eggs

Eggs are still widely consumed in the Mediterranean. Overall, less dairy products but more eggs are eaten than in the popular stereotype of the Mediterranean diet. The current guidelines in the U.S. specify up to seven eggs a week (one a day). The Mediterraneans are not counting, but my own count showed slightly more—eight to ten a week. Although we think of eggs as a breakfast food, in the Mediterranean they are more likely to be eaten for lunch or dinner, and hard-boiled eggs are the original portable snack.

The yolk is the most valued for health. Whereas some diet books still advise discarding the yolks and making an egg white omelet, traditional wisdom holds the opposite: the yolk is more valuable for health than the white.

Seafood

Everything from the sea is considered beneficial—every kind of fish and shellfish. Towns and villages even quite distant from the sea go to quite a bit of trouble to get fish and seafood. Fish cooked on the bone is more flavorful than fillets, but fillets are fine if that will increase your fish consumption.

Canned fish hold an interesting place in Mediterranean eating. In general canned food is avoided, but an important exception to this is canned fish. The use of fish preserved in olive oil in clay jars was known at least 700 years ago. Today, some of the canned fish items are considered surprisingly gourmet. Sardines, herring, anchovies, sprats, mackerel, and other smaller fish, canned in olive oil, are favored. The ones canned in water are considered less flavorful.

The smaller fish are considered safer because many environmental toxins bio-accumulate on the way up the food chain. Since smaller fish tend to be lower on oceanic food chains, any toxins in their environment have not accumulated as much.

Regarding preserved food in general, in addition to canned fish, other traditionally preserved products such as nuts, pasta, olives and pickles, and cured sausages are often used. One reason for this tradition is that in the past many times meals had to be prepared quickly because in these agricultural societies women were working in the fields right up until mealtime.

Nuts

Nuts and seeds are a surprisingly important part of the Mediterranean diet. They are a daily food—eaten as the main snack—often in the late afternoon to take the edge off hunger. They are also often eaten with fruit for dessert. Walnuts and almonds are especially favored; in the fall households usually put in a supply to last the winter. There is a folk saying that twenty almonds a day would actually sustain life for some time, as they contain so many necessary nutrients.

Pistachios in the shell are often kept as a snack. (If bowls of shelled nuts are left around to snack on, they disappear too quickly. Having to shell the pistachios at least slows things down.) Consumption is about two fairly large handfuls of nuts a day. Children under age five should not eat nuts.

Surprisingly, studies at Purdue University have shown that daily intake of this amount of nuts did not result in weight gain. The omega-3 fatty acid content of the nuts is thought to increase metabolism, and nuts contribute to steady blood sugar. In addition they are filling enough that other foods might be reduced.

If nuts and seeds are going to be a daily part of the diet, the matter of quality and freshness becomes important. Due to their fat content, rancidity is an issue for any shelled nut. Rancidty refers to the degradation of fats by exposure to light, heat, and air. Walnuts are the most susceptible to rancidity once shelled, and it can also be a problem with pine nuts. These nuts become rancid more easily in hot weather, so generally they are used only in the cooler months of the year. Transport and shelf time at the store can compromise the nuts even if you keep them under refrigeration at home.

Shelled almonds and hazelnuts, with the skin still on, do stay fresh longer than shelled walnuts. In an informal experiment I found that after three months at room temperature, whole almonds with skin intact still tasted fresh. Conversely, about sixty percent of shelled walnuts and ten percent of pecans and blanched (skinned) almonds tasted rancid.

Nuts that have been ground lose freshness quickly, so if nut meal is needed for cooking, grind it right before use in a blender or food processor. Also, avoid commercial canned nuts, which are processed at high temperatures. Sesame, pumpkin, and sunflower seeds are also popular, and are useful for those with a nut allergy.

To summarize, quality and freshness is crucial for nuts. To avoid an oxidized product, the more recently out of the shell, the better. Try shelling a few of your own nuts just to remind yourself how a fresh nut should taste. When nuts are eaten right after shelling, they can be eaten raw. Otherwise, when nuts are purchased already shelled, rancidity becomes more likely. In that case, nuts are lightly toasted. A light toasting will reduce any small trace of rancidity. However, if nuts actually taste rancid, discard them. Nuts and seeds are dry roasted without salt.

Olive Oil

The first question about oil or fat in the Mediterranean diet is not how much is taken, but rather, is it a healthy or unhealthy fat? The Mediterranean diet was traditionally at least a medium fat diet. Yet the preponderance of fats are healthy fats—usually olive oil—rather than unhealthy fats—saturated fats or, even worse, the artificial trans fats.

On the subject of the quality of fats, another consideration is how refined or processed they are. This is where extra virgin olive oil, an unrefined oil, excels. Refined seed and bean oils such as corn, sunflower, canola, and soy are often extracted with solvents and high heat. They have no defense against oxidation, and the rancidity that results is very difficult to detect.

So many commercial processed foods are made with these harmful fats that many times it is best to seek out low fat products and add your own olive oil. In other words, even those eating higher amounts of fat may request low fat foods when out of the house, because the fats found in commonly available processed foods are often harmful types.

In the traditional kitchens of the Greek islands, olive oil is used for all cooking. My own observation is that reasonable amounts of olive oil are very important to the palatability and luxurious, satisfying feeling of the Mediterranean diet. The diet has shown itself to be one of the few diets satisfying enough to stand against cravings, and a relatively high oil content is one reason.

Olive oil also seems to have solved the vegetable quandary. The slight bitterness is what is good for us about vegetables, but many do not like that taste. Olive oil and salt work to cancel out the bitter flavor.

Total fat in itself has little relation to health. Populations eating from 15 to 50 percent fat in the diet have similar rates of major disease. It is type of fat that is important. Also, total fat is not related to obesity. Dr. Willett of the Harvard School of Public Health has pointed out that if the amount of fat is reduced, the body will make certain that any calories saved will be made up for with other foods.

Trans fat is to be avoided completely, saturated fat minimized, and olive oil used in preference to the seed oils. In looking for reasons why the Mediterranean diet works for health, its ideal proportion of unsaturated fat to saturated fat is considered the most important. Beneficial dietary fats are the key to lower levels of inflammation in the body.

As the scientific evidence becomes clearer that a medium fat diet like the Mediterranean diet has better health outcomes than a low fat diet, good quality fats will become an increasingly important aspect of eating.

One way to begin is to go with the historically proven oils like olive and sesame that have kept populations healthy over thousands of years. It is interesting that as recently as ten years ago classes about the Mediterranean diet offered to those not raised on its shores assumed that it was impossible to ask people to use olive oil as their only oil or to eat several tablespoons a day. That has changed.

In concert with the notion that olive oil can replace meat and its saturated fat in generating a feeling of fullness, in the Mediterranean I noticed several levels of olive oil use. First, when a meal involves meat, already rich, very little oil is used. It then becomes more of a flavor ingredient than a basic food. For example, chicken is frequently prepared by salting it, then sauteing it for five minutes in a very minimal amount of olive oil. It is covered, cooked for twenty minutes, and then the pan is deglazed with white wine.

It is with the nonmeat dishes, such as beans and vegetables, that larger amounts of olive oil are used. These dishes often substitute for meat, thus allowing the Mediterranean diet to be a relatively low meat diet.

The choice of which olive oil to buy at the store is a personal matter of taste and budgetary constraints. No other kind of oil offers such a variety of tastes. The taste is sensitive to variety of olive, soil conditions, weather, and harvesting and milling procedure, so that with non-blended artisanal oils, no two oils are identical. Brands that have market share attempt to create some predictability from bottle to bottle by blending oils. Yet the fact remains that oil from even the same trees can vary from year to year due to weather and cultivation changes.

It is often suggested to choose a mass-market extra-virgin oil for daily cooking, and also to keep a more expensive bottle of single varietal or estate bottled extra-virgin on hand for salads. Mediterraneans believe the important point is to stick with extra-virgin and avoid the light colored oils labeled pure or simply virgin. They usually keep only one type of olive oil on hand.

To avoid being confused or intimidated by so much choice in the olive oil aisle, one way to begin is to buy at first according to budget. Then gradually extend your use to other varieties as you get more experience and begin to identify fruity, peppery, and buttery tastes.

The slight throat burn or peppery effect of some olive oils comes from the antioxidants and is a sign that the oil is fresh—and is healthy! However, olive oil is rendered much milder by cooking, which causes it to lose the distinctive olive oil taste and any peppery aftertaste. This is why it is even used for dessert cooking in the Mediterranean.

An important distinguishing characteristic of extra virgin olive oil is that it has a lower acid content. This does not so much denote a less acid taste as serve as a marker that flavor compounds are intact and not degraded. To maintain intactness after purchase, when storing olive oil, remember that it is at risk from light. An opaque bottle is the most desirable way to store it, but if not, be sure to keep the bottle in a closed cupboard, away from the heat of the stove. Don't keep it out in a clear glass cruet. Although the golden oil in a clear glass bottle illuminated by sunlight may be splendid decor, the oil as a food will be harmed by light.

In summary, the authentic Mediterranean diet is a medium fat diet. A major realization about Mediterranean diet is that a medium fat diet can be very healthy as long as it emphasizes a good fat like olive oil. In the diet, good fats, especially olive oil and nuts, replace empty sugar/starch calories and can also stand in for the satiating aspect of meat.

Dairy Products

The Mediterraneans certainly consume dairy products, yet they do so sparingly. Dairy products are used more as a garnish, a flavoring, a sprinkling. They are not really used as a meat alternative, as for example vegetarians often do in the U.S. Milk as a beverage is taken by children, but not widely used by adults.

We hear a lot about the pastoral economy of the Mediterranean, the goat milk and the shepherds. Yet, cheese-producing regions often eat little cheese themselves, preferring instead to sell it on the market. The large-scale dairy industry as we know it now is a recent phenomenon, developing with the rise of intensive animal rearing and refrigeration. That said, it is true that distinctions are made. Fresh cheeses and goat milk cheeses are considered easier to digest and less likely to make sticky artery plaque than other dairy products. Yogurt is also eaten with some frequency, but it is definitely the luxuriously thick Greek style plain yogurt.

Beans

Each Mediterranean country has its national bean dish. Each of these recipes uses olive oil and the characteristic herbs and spices of the country. It is felt that oil makes beans more digestible. Changing the soaking water one or two times also is effective.

Weekly Consumption

It appears that there is a bit of a hierarchy when it comes to animal foods. Fish and seafood are at the top, followed by eggs and organ meats. Then follows poultry—not just chicken and turkey, but duck and goose are also used. Cheese and yogurt are eaten in moderation, and red meat rarely. A typical week's menu might involve two main meals centered on fish, two on poultry, one on eggs or dairy, and two on beans or vegetables, stewed with plenty of olive oil. Red meat is used once week at most. If it is used in smaller pieces, almost as a flavoring, it can be more often.

The main issue is the amount of meat eaten per meal. If it is little, 2 to 3 ounces, then meat can be eaten more frequently. If it is a larger amount, then it is eaten less frequently.

Chapter 3. Food Choices: Vegetables and Fruits, Bread and Grains

Vegetables and Fruits

The key point about vegetables is to eat more of them, and the main concern is to make vegetables delicious so that we want to eat them. Olive oil and salt are definitely one way to make vegetables taste good. They blunt the slight bitterness that makes vegetables healthy. Take even a plain raw vegetable that does not have much appeal and marinate it in olive oil, vinegar, and salt, and it becomes a much more palatable food. Vegetables should be taken with a bit of fat, in any case, to assist in the absorption of nutrients. Cooked greens are taken with a fair amount of olive oil.

The quality of vinegar is considered important. Red wine vinegar is most often used, but the mass produced brands that have undergone accelerated aging are avoided. Balsamic vinegar is used to drizzle on fruits or cooked dishes, such as grilled vegetables, and is rarely used on salads.

One of the main food attitudes to cultivate is that vegetables are just as important as meat, and therefore just as carefully planned for and prepared. Vegetables, with olive oil to add interest and richness, are often a main dish.

If you don't like the trend towards barely cooked vegetables, cook them softer. Almost a quarter of the population has the bitter taste receptor gene that makes eating vegetables less pleasant. Increased cooking time—maybe ten minutes more—removes some of the bitterness.

Conversely, if you prefer vegetables raw, remember there is a real fondness for salads in the Mediterranean world. For most foods in the Mediterranean portion sizes are rather moderate, but in a contrast that is most apparent, salads tend to be large-sized. Travelers from other climes often note that they feel better and healthier in the

Mediterranean, and they often attribute this to the prevalence of salads.

Just like nuts, fruits are a daily, indispensable food. Juice is not common and whole fruits are preferred. Fruit is eaten at room temperature, not right out of the refrigerator. It is often eaten for dessert. Research has shown that fruit eaten at the end of a meal has benefits beyond eating fruit as a snack between meals. Fruit in the stomach thwarts the formation of harmful chemicals that are released when meat is digested. It is like the story for wine, and it is believed that both wine and fruit are better taken with meals.

Another bit of traditional wisdom is that meals should always have a liquid aspect. In cool weather, soups often fulfill this, and in hot weather, the liquid aspect is provided by salads and fresh fruit.

Two to three pieces of fruit a day are eaten. Quality is paramount. Purely as a matter of flavor, this is one case where organic might more nearly mimic the quality found in the Mediterranean.

When fruit is brought to the table for dessert, it is not the proverbial big bowl of fruit—it is much more likely to be already peeled and cut up—in a most user-friendly form.

Dessert is thus more likely to be what could be called "regular foods"—fruit, nuts, and/or cheese— rather than being a sweet. The epitome of this is the custom of the thirteen desserts of the Christmas season. This is made up of four fresh fruits, four dry fruits, four kinds of nuts, and almond nougat.

Bread and Grains

The general rule about grain consumption is that it varies according to activity level. It helps to get some historical and cross-cultural perspective on this. The dense carbohydrates of grain are primarily an energy source, so the more physical activity and manual labor engaged in, the more grain was eaten. Historically, in the Mediterranean, both men and women who did agricultural and household labor ate large quantities of bread. Bread could easily be half a meal in terms of physical amount.

But even in the past, bread consumption varied by occupational status, with those in sedentary occupations eating less. In many countries bread came in a 6 pound round loaf, and typical consumption was three pounds a day for those doing physical labor and one pound a day for sedentary work. Today, when far fewer are employed in physical labor and incomes are higher, bread consumption has fallen dramatically in the Mediterranean world. Surveys show that bread consumption is less than half that of forty years ago. Other cultures have also followed this pattern. In China, six bowls of rice per meal was the standard amount for physical laborers. In Mexico, a laboring man ate up to twenty tortillas in a meal. In both countries, grain consumption has now decreased.

Incomes were also always a crucial factor in higher consumption, as the staff of life was purposely kept inexpensive. Mediterranean governments often controlled or subsidized the price of bread to avoid actual hunger or political unrest. But over time, as incomes increased in many countries, bread assumed a lesser role in the meal as more variety appeared on the plate. The light baguette type often replaced the substantial whole grain country bread, which could literally be a meal in itself.

In spite of reduced consumption, bread still occupies a very special place in the Mediterranean world, in daily life and daily conversation. There are many folk and religious customs involving bread, and a defining change of modern life was when families stopped grinding wheat and baking bread weekly in their own beehive ovens.

Bread has entered the ancestral memory as the all-important famine food—literally the staff of life. First, grain can be stored and eaten when other crops have failed. Just as important, I was told repeatedly by people who had endured famine as recently as World War II, bread soaked in olive oil was the only available food that could sate one's appetite and leave one free from gnawing hunger, a role performed in times of plenty by animal foods.

Bread is still eaten daily, and it is considered a basic, balancing food. But it is eaten in less quantity nowadays. There are myriad stories about how in older times travelers to northern Europe from the Mediterranean were shocked by how little bread was served with meals. The solitary roll of the north seemed completely inadequate compared to the heaped-up bread baskets of the south. However, in a sign of the changing consumption pattern, today the equivalent of a single roll often suffices in Mediterranean tavernas. Mainly it is at working men's and laborers' restaurants that one still sees the bread piled high. Students and young people, those with active jobs, those active in sports, or anyone with increased caloric requirements can eat more grains. Meanwhile, the more sedentary cut back.

In the Mediterranean, the fresher the bread, the better—it does not retain top flavor beyond one day. Bakers grind flour fresh daily, and bread is shopped for daily, six days a week. The bread seems to suit the food well and seems to be formulated to go particularly well with olive oil and olive oil sauces: its texture is suited for sopping up the oil. Sourdough bread is the norm, and soft bread is not appreciated.

Chapter 4. Beverages: Coffee, Wine, and Water

Coffee and Wine

Coffee is considered a physical, mental, and mood tonic, taken in small amounts. I got the impression that the two beverages considered tonic, coffee and wine, are used to modulate mood and alertness. Coffee is taken in the morning, because liquids should be emphasized early in the day. Another cup might be taken later during the day or after a meal in order to maintain alertness. Then, in the evening, a glass of wine accompanies and enhances dinner.

Drinking habits are considered to be directly related to eating habits. Filling up the stomach rapidly, even with plain water, translates into eating more. Thus, sipping beverages is cultivated as a way to train oneself to also eat slowly and moderately.

Caffeine has recently been shown to have benefits ranging from increased cognition and increased glucose tolerance to elevated mood. However, some people have caffeine sensitivity and should take very little or none at all. Even without the sensitivity, it is notable that in the Mediterranean it is used with moderation. Too much caffeine can affect sleep, and sleep is just as important a tonic as coffee.

In the Mediterranean, coffee tends to be served with a glass of water, which is taken after the coffee. This is considered to counteract any negative effects from caffeine or acidity. Also, ground coffee is often mixed with 15% ground, roast chicory before brewing (as in the New Orleans fashion), as this also reduces acidity.

Coffee on an empty stomach, as in that first cup in the morning before breakfast, is cautioned against. This traditional wisdom may be valid, as studies have indicated that coffee on an empty stomach often raises blood sugar.

Finally, coffee in moderation is considered to be an appetite suppressant.

Regarding wine, the key issue is moderation. The amount of wine matters tremendously. And the crucial point about this is that wine and beer are regarded as foods and are taken with other foods. Also, many times wine is mixed with water or sparkling water—this is seen as a sign of how serious one is about moderating consumption. For wines that are not mixed, care is taken to sip a glass of water along with the wine.

In the most basic sense, wine is not an instrument of intoxication. Indeed, drinking wine is seen as an opportunity to practice the golden mean and to put the art of good living into practice. Wine lightens the tongue and lubricates social interaction around the table. Relaxation at the table is considered important, and wine can add to the relaxed spirit. It is felt that moderation in drinking wine extends out to other parts of life.

The alcohol content of wine is more variable than it used to be. Many present-day wines tend to have more alcohol or higher proof than before, as the grapes are left on the vine longer to develop more flavor. New types of yeast have also raised the alcohol content of some wines. This calls for more caution in consumption, as any benefits of alcohol are dose dependent, and more is not necessarily better. In order to imbibe while reducing the effect, one key is to not have that glass of wine at happy hour or as an aperitif before dinner, but to wait until one is a few bites into the meal.

Children are introduced in the family setting to wine (watered) at a relatively young age, and this is thought to reduce the incidence of alcoholism and binge drinking later. Yet, that might depend on the whole culture reinforcing the message that the role of wine is not as a means of intoxication.

Alcoholics, pregnant women, people taking certain medications, and people with liver problems should not drink even wine. My own observations showed that with wine, men and older people took more: the culture considers it a tonic that has the most benefit for men over forty. In line with what is recommended, I observed that men averaged about a cup a day. Women took a few sips of wine at meals, adding up to perhaps one to two cups of wine per week.

Coffee and wine are at base happiness tonics. If you don't see them that way—if either make you feel you are hooked or if for you they are health problems—then it is best to refrain. The beverages have some positive and some negative effects, and it depends on the individual which is most germane.

Water

Mediterraneans do seem to drink more water, and good tasting and good quality water is highly valued. Drinking enough water is not something that is left to chance. The principle about water is that it must be made inviting to the individual in order to drink enough of it. Do what is necessary to make your water attractive and inviting to you. Rather than forcing yourself to drink, make the water more enticing. Make it cooler, warmer, more available, add lemon, lime, or carbonation, or filter it. Do not sweeten it, however. Make it easily accessible—in the Mediterranean a pitcher of water is on the table at every meal.

Thirst is not always a reliable guide—the sensation of thirst is easily trained away. If you find it inconvenient to drink, you can train yourself not to notice thirst. The mechanism of thirst also is less reliable in cool weather, and studies have shown that we are more likely to become dehydrated in winter than in summer. Yet the studies concluded that the number of cups of liquid to drink is not uniform—it depends on activity level, the weather, humidity of indoor air, body size, and how much liquid is in the food.

An old proverb says: drink before meals to lose weight; drink after meals to gain weight. Old sayings also support the idea that drinking hot water first thing every morning upon arising is rejuvenating. Conversely, ice-cold beverages with meals are thought to retard digestion and encourage faster eating of larger quantities. Even in hot weather it is considered important to take beverages out of refrigeration a few minutes before drinking them to take the edge off the extreme cold.

Chapter 5. Tips and Attitudes

Honey

A pound of honey represents many thousands of flights by bees between flower and hive. Maybe this is why Mediterraneans don't agree with the often-heard notion that honey is just the same as sugar insofar as it affects the body. Honey has anti-inflammatory and immunity-boosting properties.

Raw is best, and as much as two teaspoons a day are taken. Interestingly, if a teaspoon of honey is taken in the morning followed by a cup of tea or of warm water, this is considered to raise the metabolism and encourage gradual weight loss. Children under one year should not eat honey.

Superfoods

Olive oil and wine are considered the real superfoods of the Mediterranean diet, possibly because they reduce oxidation. The Mediterraneans themselves attribute longevity to these two foods.

It is also pointed out that an additional virtue of olive oil is that it goes so well with other healthy foods like fish, beans, and vegetables, and so increases the likelihood of eating and enjoying them.

In addition, another suggestion is that it is considered anti-aging to take one heaping teaspoon of tahini in the morning before breakfast, followed by a glass of water. For those without nut allergies, 6 to 8 pine nuts a day are recommended. A small amount (about one ounce) of dark chocolate (70% cacao or over) is also considered a tonic food.

Salt in Cooking

Salt is used this way in cooking: the amount of salt to be used is divided in two and half added at the beginning of cooking and the other half towards the end. This leads to a more complex flavor. Sea salt is used.

Dressing a Salad

The key to a good green salad is to toss it very well and combine it thoroughly with the dressing, not just pour the dressing on top. When using raw onions in a salad, cut the onions from top to bottom rather than through the equator. This increases the sweet flavor and decreases the bite.

Ripeness of Fruits and Vegetables

The point of vine- and tree-ripened is that many nutrients come the last few days of ripening. In addition they taste so much better that they can actually compete with a sweet.

Fruits that are fully ripe when purchased will spoil much more quickly, though. That is how it should be, as a belief in the Mediterranean is that foods with long shelf life don't nourish—if bacteria aren't interested, our cells probably aren't either.

A food writer once described her experience of cooking in the Mediterranean as that of racing decay. Before her very eyes the newly bought fruits would begin to sprout mold the minute she got them home from market, as things are picked much riper and don't have as long a shelf life before they must be used. This can be controlled now with refrigeration, but the principle is still that long shelf life is not really desirable.

Many fruits, including peaches, melons, grapes, and apples, must ripen on the tree. Once picked they do not ripen further, but only soften.

Enough Time

Rushing through meals or not giving time and attention to what one is consuming is considered a red-flag danger point. This slow food culture is given far more emphasis in the Mediterranean than in other parts of the world. The one certainty is that we must put time into our eating. It is a matter of values, but in addition longer meals slow the absorption of sugars and fats and leave time for the production of digestive enzymes.

Regular Mealtimes/Portable Snacks

It is considered crucial to not allow yourself to become too hungry. Once a state of excessive hunger is reached, all bets are off as they say. In the Mediterranean, this is handled by regular meal times that are stuck to through thick and thin. If we don't have this stability in our fast-paced life, we must substitute planning and ingenuity. For example, if you might be stranded where good food is not readily available, carry food with you. Many foods in the Mediterranean diet are readily portable. Hard boiled eggs, fruit, nuts, and celery and carrot sticks are especially used.

Olives and Sweets

A proverb instructs that to overcome a craving for sweets, eat olives.

Adjusting for the Season

Seasonal eating implies, in addition to emphasizing foods in season, also eating more grains and vegetables in the summer, and more fat and protein in the winter. The first fruits or vegetables of the season are considered especially nutritious, and end-of-season or stored produce less so. A proverb puts it, "eat young vegetables to stay young."

Seasonal eating also applies to breakfast. The Mediterranean breakfast can be light, one reason being that dinner is often eaten very late. However, this pattern of late dinner and light breakfast is mainly a summer pattern. In winter, breakfast is a more substantial meal.

It is believed best to wait until one is hungry to eat in the morning. Until then, the important point is to rehydrate and drink plenty of fluids in the morning.

Small Changes

Even small changes in a positive direction are considered important. Incremental changes do add up when they are done almost every day.

Finding Ways to Enjoy Shopping for Fresh Foods

The question of food choices starts outside the kitchen, at the market. Supermarkets have plenty of real food, but this has to be sought, as supermarkets are also loaded with fake foods.

Give time and attention to your food shopping. Ask what you can do to make shopping more satisfying for yourself. Time is a major factor—less rushed shopping is more pleasurable. If you don't like crowds, go early or late. If part of the pleasure is finding good value, shop the sales on fruits and vegetables.

For all the dissatisfaction with the American food system, at this very moment there is a huge amount of beautiful yet economical food already in the marketplace, just waiting for us. We need to know how to find it and choose it, and organize ourselves to do so.

The Golden Mean

The Mediterranean diet is a medium fat diet, which avoids the problem of many low fat diets that they are not satisfying to the palate or body without an inordinate increase in the proportion of carbohydrates.

Those with intolerance to oil can eat the diet as a low fat diet by altering recipes and will still receive many benefits. However, the authentic Mediterranean diet avoids extremes and is a medium fat diet employing at least 3 or 4 tablespoons of oil a day.

In the same way, the Mediterranean diet avoids going to the extreme of completely excluding red meat or dairy foods; it merely recommends much more moderate amounts of these foods than is typical of many diets in the U.S.

This avoidance of the extreme is a well-known value from ancient times in the Mediterranean, not just in their dietary recommendations but in many parts of life. It can be seen again in their emphasis on consuming moderate amounts of wine or coffee, rather than either complete prohibition or indulgence. The "golden mean" could be considered the essence of their traditional wisdom. In making changes in diet or activity level, don't be too radical—start with little changes—but be persistent.

Preciousness of Food

It is a saying in the Mediterranean that both food and sleep are surpassingly sweeter after toil. Most of us living in modern developed countries may never really get back to that fundamental realization, but I do believe that in the coming years the preciousness of food will be reestablished. With the coming resource pressures, no longer will we forget where our food comes from or waste a third of our food. Along with the Mediterraneans, we will know that food is the central axis of life. If we get eating right, other parts of life more easily fall into place.

Chapter 6. Exercise and Sleep

Exercise

The evolution of human society has been away from physical effort and towards ease. This now has reached a point of diminishing returns. As physical activity is increasingly engineered out of our everyday life, the approach taken in the Mediterranean is to try to make exercise as natural a part of daily life as possible. Indeed, it is thought that the body intuitively tends to rebel against exercise not connected with otherwise purposeful activity. This is because for our early ancestors, pointless or wasted energy expenditure was something to be avoided at all costs.

Thus, exercise is approached through gardening and housework, possibly without major labor saving appliances, through taking the stairs and walking whenever feasible, even by chopping wood.

Another tack taken is to multitask after a fashion: walking time is also a social time if done with others. In the Mediterranean there is the traditional paseo (a promenade at sunset in the town square). Walking can be combined with birdwatching, meditation, or music listening. There are virtual workouts online that are shared with others.

One important factor often mentioned in the Mediterranean is that, unless ill, one should be on one's feet a minimum of two to three hours a day. It would seem easy enough to be standing that long, and sales, nursing, and assembly line personnel definitely do at work. However, studies have shown that those with desk jobs, and even many youth in this computer and TV age, do not spend enough time on their feet. Interestingly, I observed on Skyros Island a personal discipline undertaken by many residents that addressed the question of standing. They kept themselves busy with tasks and consciously did not allow themselves to sit down from morning waking time until 12 noon. Sitting was something to be earned.

The goal is to be an active person—it has been pointed out that exercise can actually be negative if the exerciser believes they are absolved from being a generally active person. Research has shown that even incidental movement is important, as it is uninterrupted periods of sitting down that are to be avoided. One easy way to begin is to stand up and take a stretch once an hour. A standup desk is useful for the desk bound. Another possibility is to purposefully avoid some modern conveniences that have made life unnecessarily sedentary.

The good news about exercise is that even the smallest bits of activity count. Just a little physical activity can make a difference; it is not all or nothing. Like eating habits, exercise habits are an area where incremental changes can accumulate impressively over time.

Sleep

Mediterraneans are renowned for their characteristic style of sleep, including the infamous afternoon siesta. Their sleep is split into two discrete time periods, night sleep and siesta afternoon sleep. Sleep researchers have called this bimodal or bifurcated sleep.

Knowing that this is the norm in the Mediterranean can bring a feeling of relief to those who find they cannot go to bed every night and sleep straight through for eight hours. There is more than one way to sleep. It has been theorized that bimodal sleep was normal for humans before the invention of electricity and artificial light. During the long winter nights, before artificial light, there might be two periods of sleep separated by a time of wakefulness. In summer, people awoke very early for agricultural labor and then napped in the heat of the day.

Split sleep in the Mediterranean is a result of climate and architecture. In the late afternoon the thick walled houses begin to radiate the heat absorbed from the sun during the day. By evening they start to seem unbearably hot and remain so until well after midnight.

This may be the source of the well-known "going out every night" culture and the late hours of the Mediterranean. In some countries, such as in Spain, the people dine as late as 11 PM, and bedtime can be 2 AM or later. Split working hours and a siesta from 3 to 5 PM compensate.

Another consideration is that Mediterranean houses have thick, working shutters. This is thought to be a necessity, since, if one is to sleep during the day, it is considered crucial to sleep in complete darkness. Interior sources of light, such as electronic equipment or illuminated clocks, are extinguished.

It is considered important to air out the bed every morning. The bed is not made immediately, but the quilts are laid back for several hours.

If there are sleep difficulties or insomnia, the first suggestion is to consolidate sleep by decreasing or limiting the time in bed. However, where there is no insomnia, light sleep or dozing is thought to have its own value. It may not be quite as rejuvenating as deep sleep, but it is restful, enjoyable, and to be appreciated in itself. Relax, allow yourself to doze, and receive the benefits of your light sleep.

Chapter 7. Quick Start

Here are some ways to start right away:

Use olive oil

Eat both a cooked vegetable and a salad at meals

Eat a few pieces of whole fruit (not juice) every day

Eat a couple of snacks of nuts every day

Eat smaller portions of meat

Eat beans several times a week

Eat an occasional vegetarian entrée

Chapter 8. Three Mediterranean Ideas for Life Satisfaction

Mediterranean ideas about how to live are a deep subject indeed. Visitors to the area are often struck by the distinctive quality of the outlook on life. They feel they are reminded anew of what is really important in life.

Many aspects of the Mediterranean way of life do stand as a certain challenge to the whole current and direction of modern life. This is valuable in that it allows us to re-access our own ideas.

One critical factor that lies at the base of the outlook is the celebrated Mediterranean love of life in all its guises. This love of life stresses its eternally and boisterously flowing nature; life is endlessly creating, embellishing, and self-renewing. Obstruction or stultification of the unfolding is to be avoided as both wrongheaded and futile. Added to this is the strong realization of how easily this can happen and how easily humans can be pushed off course.

I will choose only three themes about life satisfaction and aim only to give a little food for thought regarding these profound subjects.

The First Idea for Life Satisfaction: Combat Time Poverty

The time poverty of modern life has an economic basis, but it is one of the harshest circumstances of our times. Recognize its inhuman aspects and counter it as much as possible. Although we are taught to do more, sometimes do less. Remove items from the to do list; this will leave more room for the important things. These "important things" have a tendency to require that we demonstrate patience. They withdraw under our rush and are not about to compete for our time.

One of the most frequent factors adding to time pressure is high expectations. Give up the search for perfection. Too high expectations can especially be a trap in relationships.

Children growing up in a time pressed environment are thought to particularly suffer.

The Second Idea for Life Satisfaction: Keep Human Scale

One of the most universal observations about Mediterranean cultures is that regimentation is intensely disliked. Indeed, many have observed that sabotaging and defeating regimentation is central to the whole way of life.

Large-scale systems are seen as a breeding ground of regimentation and are also questioned. Their inexorable quality, the inability to reform or dislodge them once established, result in the question of scale often becoming a question of power. Individuals feel, and often are, powerless when faced with large-scale systems.

Human scale is beloved. Keep it wherever possible and question bringing more and more parts of life into a systems-centered realm. In those areas where large scale is useful, inform it by ways to maintain flexibility and attention to individual needs.

Another aspect of keeping human life as the measure is the Mediterranean advice to get out and experience life rather than letting media and devices do all the work for you. One concern is that if the actual world becomes less livable over time, there will be more temptation to spend time in a virtual world. Another concern is that a synthetically created reality can exert greater emotional power than concrete actuality, increasing the inclination to convert real life into digital life.

The Third Idea for Life Satisfaction: Beware of Infringing Natural Laws for Long Periods

Nature may be fooled for a short time, but not for a long time. With this last idea we approach the subject of health and food yet again. We have mentioned that both continuous sitting and artificial exercise infringe the natural laws of the body. In the area of food, an analogy would be the continuous availability of hyperpalatable foods. What are called hyperpalatable foods are ones that will be eaten even when one is not hungry.

These foods, often sweets, traditionally have been only occasional treats, due to expense and cultural limits on when they would be eaten. The current global dilemma is that food industries, in response to an ancient human dream, have made these foods both cheap and continually available.

This seems like the fulfillment of the age old human dream of a universal utopia of abundance, but all over the world it has been found that it leads invariably to significant overeating and consequent problems. The body's appetite mechanism is not meant to be overthrown in this manner. Yet it is happening worldwide on a very large scale—human nature finds it an offer too good to pass up.

How can we keep from infringing natural laws? Let's get to know ways of life inspired by traditions that have provided satisfaction for thousands of years. Let's get to know the Mediterranean diet and use it to make our life better.

Chapter 9. Recipes

Home Cooking in the Mediterranean

The home cooking that I experienced in the Mediterranean was simple, honest, and straight-forward. Because of its simplicity, the basic structure of a dish can be easily comprehended. The ingredients for each dish are few. The basic flavor ingredients are olive oil, salt, and often lemon juice. It's surprising how dishes made from simple building blocks can be so delicious and fulfilling.

Many worthy cookbooks exist for Mediterranean cuisine (several mentioned in the suggestions for further reading in the back of the book), and new ones appear regularly. However, some of the recipes or techniques I encountered are not well covered in the cookbook literature, and I present them here.

Some of the simpler dishes I have expressed as if talking to a friend, as they were expressed to me. For those with more ingredients, I have listed them at the top in the standard way.

* * * * * * * *

Mediterranean Fish Soup

This is a main course.

2 small zucchini, cut into sticks	½ C flat leafed parsley, chopped
2 carrots, cut into sticks	½ C olive oil
1 large onion, cut into small chunks	2½ C water
1 potato, cut into chunks	salt and pepper, to taste
2 stalks celery, with leaves if possible	1 lb white fish fillets, preferably cod
	lemon wedges

Put all of the ingredients except fish and lemon in a pot, bring to boil, then turn down heat and simmer for 15 minutes. Add white fish fillets. Mediterranean cod was traditionally used, but any firm white fish serves well. Cook at a slow simmer for 12 minutes, never boiling. Serve with fresh lemon to squeeze into the soup.

Lemon Chicken

I have found that an electric slow cooker can be used for recipes calling for cooking on the hearth in the embers of a fire, which is a method often used in the Mediterranean. The long, slow cooking develops the meltingly tender textures and deep flavors that characterize Mediterranean cooking. (Of course, grilling is used when shorter cooking times are desired.)

Chicken pieces with bone in would be used as meats and fish are thought to be more succulent and flavorful if cooked with bone in. A similar idea applies to many other foods. For example, olives retain their flavor better with the pit in place.

Mediterranean chicken has less fat so it would be cooked with the skin. With our higher fat chickens, skinless can be used.

This chicken dish can be made in a slow cooker or on the stovetop.

Slow Cooker

Place a cut up skinless chicken into the slow cooker. Sprinkle with salt and oregano, add 1 sliced onion, 1 cup lemon juice, and ½ cup olive oil. Cook on high setting for 2 hours and low setting for 6 to 8 hours.

Stove Top

Place the above ingredients plus 2 tablespoons water in a heavy pot. Bring to a boil over medium heat and boil for 2 minutes. Cover, turn heat down low and simmer for 30 minutes, checking a few times to see if more water needs to be added.

Bean Cooking

These are the directions I received in a Skyros Island kitchen and they produce delicious beans.

Soak cannellini or other white beans overnight or for 8 hours. Do not leave beans soaking for much more than 8 to 10 hours or they lose flavor. Drain and place in a heavy pot. For ½ pound dry beans, add ½ cup olive oil, ½ t salt, ½ t pepper, and 3 crushed cloves of fresh garlic. Pour on 3 cups of water and bring to a boil. Reduce flame to low and cook for 2 hours minimum up to 4 hours, adding more water as needed.

Lentil Soup

This is a classic "better the next day" soup, so a lot is made at once. It even improves if it is "twice cooked." That is, the second day add more water and simmer for 20 more minutes. The lentils become velvety in texture.

1 lb lentils

1 big onion or 2

  small onions,

  chopped

3 celery stalks,

  sliced thin

1 natural stock or

  cube of bouillon,

  any flavor

5 C water

6 tablespoons olive oil

1 teaspoon salt

1 tomato, chopped

2 tablespoons tomato

  paste

Put all ingredients in a large stock pot, bring to a boil, and simmer, covered, for 30 minutes.

Note: Stock cubes or powder are often used to enrich bean dishes in the Mediterranean.

As a variation, this soup is also made using black beans.

Cinnamon Toast with Olive Oil

Olive oil loses its distinctive taste when it is heated, and it is often used in sweets. Try this to see.

4 slices whole grain
  bread
4 tablespoons honey,
  with a few drops of water
  added so it spreads easily

4 tablespoons olive oil
4 teaspoons ground
  cinnamon

Put bread on a flat cookie sheet and drizzle each slice with 1 tablespoon olive oil. Broil 6 inches from the broiling element for 3 minutes. Remove from oven and spread the honey on the face-up side of each slice. Sprinkle with cinnamon. Return to the broiler for one minute. Serve immediately while hot.

A Popular Snack

Place a slice of whole grain bread on a plate. Drizzle it with olive oil to taste—at least several teaspoons. Sprinkle it with oregano, rosemary, thyme, and 1 clove garlic, minced. Further sprinkle it with black olive freshly sliced off the pit and walnut pieces in winter, or diced fresh ripe tomato in summer. Bake in a 300 degree oven (no need to preheat) for 8 minutes.

How to Serve Tahini

Tahini is generally mixed to a creamy texture with water before serving. Put ½ cup tahini in a bowl. Beat it well—beating improves the flavor of tahini. Then add ¼ cup water and mix well. At first, the water will seem not to be mixing well with the tahini, but continue mixing and it will become very smooth. A pinch of salt and the juice of half a lemon is often added.

Another way of serving tahini is to mix it with honey. Instead of becoming creamy, as when mixed with water, the tahini thickens. Good quality and good tasting honey is important. The proportion is about ¼ cup honey to 1 cup tahini. Mix them thoroughly. Often, lightly toasted walnuts are mixed in, and the mixture is formed into a roll with wax paper and sliced.

Toasted Hazelnuts

Hazelnuts, or filberts, are one of the best eating nuts. They often seem underappreciated, although among other virtues they are considered more digestible than almonds.

Roast a half pound of hazelnuts in a 300 degree oven for 20 to 25 minutes, depending on their size. Place them in a tea towel and rub off the skins. Let the nuts cool, and rub one more time in the tea towel. A little skin will remain, as it is difficult to remove completely.

Tender Eggs

These eggs are cooked longer than soft boiled, but less than hard boiled; they are tender. They are often drizzled with olive oil and sprinkled with a tiny bit of celery salt, which is thought to go well with eggs. Bring eggs to boil, starting with cold water, and boil for 30 seconds. Turn off heat, cover, and leave in the water for 6 minutes before draining.

Ariani Drink

1 C yogurt, plain	1 tablespoon honey
½ C water, or more	juice of ½ lemon
to taste	

Mix in blender, or whip very well by hand. A variation is to add ¼ C grape juice.

Fruit

Raw fruit is most often served on platters, already prepared and cut up into bite size pieces, ready to eat. Often the peeling and cutting are done at the table, though, after the meal while talking continues. One person can take charge, or if there are enough knives, everyone can peel and cut their own. Often two types of fruit are served. Everyone has their own smaller plate and fork, and they take as much or little as they wish. In addition, prearranged fruit desserts, like the following, are appreciated.

Peaches in Watermelon Juice

½ small watermelon   4 ripe peaches

  or ¼ large one

Make watermelon juice by pureeing watermelon chunks in a blender or food processor, then straining through a colander. Or, lacking a blender, set watermelon chunks in a colander that is then placed in a bowl, and mash the watermelon with a potato masher. Peel the peaches and cut them into bite size chunks. Chill the peaches in the watermelon juice for one hour or more. This is a cooling and refreshing summer dessert.

Melon with Port Wine

2 cantaloupes   1 C port wine

Halve the cantaloupes and remove the seeds. With a fork, jab holes into the flesh of each cantaloupe half. Be careful not to pierce the outer rind. Pour ¼ C port into each half and swirl around so the wine enters the holes. Cover and marinate for 4 hours. Drain (the wine can be reused) and serve.

Figs and Yogurt

Marinate fresh figs in orange juice for 1 hour in the refrigerator. Mix ½ cup of the orange juice into 1 cup Greek style yogurt. Put the yogurt into bowls, and top with the figs, sliced. Sprinkle with pistachio nuts. With the few nuts needed (about 6 per serving), you can shell them yourself rather than buying shelled pistachio nuts, which aren't as fresh.

Simple Berry Dessert

Limoncello is a lemon liqueur with a full, ripe lemon flavor. This liqueur pairs well with fruit—a few drops sprinkled over fruit complements the flavor. Additionally, studies have shown that adding alcohol to fruits helps increase the antioxidant activity of the fruits.

Wash and halve 1 pint strawberries, or use ½ strawberries and ½ blueberries. Sprinkle 4 tablespoons Limoncello over the berries. Fully ripe strawberries are sweet enough, but if more sweetness is needed, sprinkle with 1 teaspoon sugar. Let sit in the refrigerator for 1 hour. Mash slightly and serve.

Further Reading

Acquista, Angelo, *The Mediterranean Prescription*. NY: Ballantine Books, 2006.

Brennan, Georgeanne, *Olives, Anchovies, and Capers: the Secret Ingredients of the Mediterranean Table*. San Francisco: Chronicle Books, 2001.

Culinary Institute of America, *Mediterranean Cooking with the Culinary Institute of America*. Hoboken, NJ: John Wiley, 2013.

Ferguson, Claire, *Extra Virgin: Cooking With Olive Oil*. NY: Ryland, 2000.

Fisher, M.F.K., "Two Kitchens in Provence" in *As They Were*. NY: Vintage, 1983.

Gordon, Jonas and Sandra Gordon, *30 Secrets of the World's Healthiest Cuisines*. NY: Wiley, 2000.

Gray, Patience, *Honey From a Weed*. NY: Harper and Row, 1987.

Jenkins, Nancy Harmon, *The New Mediterranean Diet Cookbook*. NY: Bantam, 2009. Includes Appendix I: "The Mediterranean Diet and Health" by Antonia Trichopoulou and Dimitri Trichopoulou.

Also, the Mediterranean diet and its scientific basis are regularly covered by several newsletters including the *Tufts University Health and Nutrition Letter, Harvard Health Letter,* and *Berkeley Wellness Letter*. All have keyword search at the top of their web pages. Enter the search term "Mediterranean diet."

Jenkins, Sara and Mindy Fox, *Olives and Oranges*. NY: Houghton Mifflin, 2008.

Kazantzakis, Nikos, *Zorba the Greek*. NY: Simon and Schuster, 1981.

Krasner, Deborah, *The Flavors of Olive Oil: A Tasting Guide and Cookbook*. NY: Simon and Schuster, 2002.

Kremezi, Aglaia and Martin Brigdale, *The Mediterranean Pantry*. NY: Artisan, 1994.

Louv, Richard, *The Nature Principle: Reconnecting With Life in a Virtual Age*. Chapel Hill: Algonquin, 2012.

McCartney, Paul, Stella and Mary, *The Meat Free Monday Cookbook*. NY: Kyle, 2012.

Rosenblum, Mort, *Olives, The Life and Lore of a Noble Fruit*. NY: North Point, 1996.

Seaver, Jeannette, *My New Mediterranean Cookbook: Eat Better, Live Longer by Following the Mediterranean Diet.* NY: Arcade, 2004.

Shulman, Martha Rose, *Mediterranean Light: Delicious Recipes from the World's Healthiest Cuisine.* NY: Bantam, 1989.

Simon, Harvey, *The No Sweat Exercise Plan.* NY: McGraw-Hill, 2006.

Small, Gary and Gigi Vorgan, *iBrain: Surviving the Technological Alteration of the Human Brain.* NY: Harper Collins, 2008.

Weir, Joanne, *From Tapas to Meze.* NY: Crown, 1994.

Wolfert, Paula, *The Slow Mediterranean Kitchen.* Hoboken, NJ: Wiley, 2003.

Wright, Clifford, *A Mediterranean Feast: The Story of the Birth of the Celebrated Cuisines of the Mediterranean.* NY: William Morrow, 1999.

www.ingramcontent.com/pod-product-compliance
Lightning Source LLC
Chambersburg PA
CBHW060423290526
45791CB00002B/855